How to Improve Your Memory:

Overcoming Poor Recall

Using Simple Memory Exercises

Phillip P. Burrell

Copyright © 2011 Phillip P. Burrell
All Rights Reserved.

Reproduction or translation of any part of this work beyond that permitted by section 107 or 108 of the 1976 United States Copyright Act without permission of the copyright owner is unlawful. Requests for permission or further information should be addressed to the author.

This publication is designed to provide accurate and authoritative information in regard to the subject matter covered. It is sold the understanding that the publisher is not engaged in rendering medical services. If medical advice or other expert assistance is required, the services of a competent professional person should be sought.

First Printing, 2011

ISBN: 978-1460923016

Printed in the United States of America

Dedication

For those struggling
to remember

"Memory is the mother of all wisdom."
Aeschylus

Table of Contents

Chapter 1 9

Our Magnificent Memory 9

Chapter 2 15

Understanding Memory Functions 15

Chapter 3 21

Human Memory Myths 21

Chapter 4 27

Memory Busters 27

Chapter 5 37

Boosting Memory From Within 37

Chapter 6 43

How Diet Can Help Your Brain 43

Chapter 7 53

Memory Solutions 53

Chapter 8 57

Sharpening Your Five Senses 57

Chapter 9 67

Brain Workouts 67

Chapter 10 73

Memory Improvement Strategies........................... 73

Chapter 11 87

Beating Absentmindedness 87

Chapter 12 93

Acing Those Exams 93

Chapter 1

Our Magnificent Memory

> *"Yesterday's just a memory, tomorrow is never what it's supposed to be."*
>
> **Bob Dylan**

The human memory is one of man's most important tools used to survive in modern society. In the ultra-competitive world that we now tread, having a poor memory can equate to having an extremely difficult time in school or at work.

We need to have good memory to handle the information overload that is characteristic of our day and age. Whether a person is a poet, artist, accountant or businessperson, he still needs good memory to respond to life's daily demands.

Since you are reading this book, we are going to assume that you have experienced poor recall and this might have possibly been a source of distress for you. Having poor recall may have also prevented you from excelling at work or at school.

If you have ever been embarrassed or extremely saddened by poor memory, it is time to smile once more, because contained within this book are the holistic solutions that will help you improve your memory by addressing this complex problem in its entirety.

The Nature of Human Memory

When a person is born, he has already been equipped with everything he needs to develop an excellent memory that should serve him well past his prime.

So if you have poor recall *now*, that simply means that you were not able to exert the right type of effort to improve your memory before. This also means that the time is ripe to maximize your use of your own memory.

But before we can do that, we must understand *what memory is* in the first place.

We can liken the human memory to a dynamic, enormous data bank that analyzes and stores all forms of stimuli during our waking and sleeping moments. The human memory is so efficient that you can actually train yourself to remember a significant portion of what you dream of at night.

The human brain constantly receives stimuli of all forms during our waking hours.

It is responsible for making sound decisions and is also responsible for *remembering*. The task of handling all the functions that are required of the human brain is handled by billions of brain cells. Brain cells are not only capable of communicating with one another, but with the other various systems that keep the human body running smoothly as well.

The brain may well be the most important organ in the human body. Without it, all organ and organ systems would shut down.

Because of its numerous functions, it requires a large amount of oxygen. It consumes an estimated *twenty percent* of the total oxygen gained by the body during respiration, which is also why a person who is *deprived* of oxygen for a few minutes is already considered in peril.

Before we delve into memory improvement techniques, we must first establish a baseline or theoretical foundation about memory itself. So what *is* human memory? In a nutshell, memory is the capacity of the human brain to receive, store and *recall* information about the world we live in.

Memory is by no means secondary to other conscious brain functions. Without a functional memory, a person would not be able to *learn* anything. And without learning, human life would be extremely limited.

Now, one must not confuse the entirety of human memory with one of its most well-known sub functions – recall. A group of people can have healthy, normal brains but they will have varying capacities to recall information. What accounts for this variation between individuals?

The difference lies in the way we *hone* recall – because recalling any kind of information is actually a *skill* that can be learned and improved continually.

There is no age limit to this. Whether you are 25 or 75, you can still take the steps to improve your memory. The only obstacle perhaps is one's *drive* (or the lack of it) to succeed in improving one's memory.

However, if you are the type who likes overnight results, you may be disappointed since no effective memory improvement technique works overnight.

But if you want an approach to memory improvement that will serve you for the long-term, you have come to the right place. This book is all about long-term memory improvement that you can use to enhance every aspect of your life from school, work, and of course, daily living.

Chapter 2

Understanding Memory Functions

> *"You never know when you're making a memory."*
>
> **Rickie Lee Jones**

Not all memories are equal. For the human memory system to work efficiently, the human brain 'categorizes' memories into three sub-types: *short-term*, *long-term* and *sensory*. To understand *how* we store memories, we must understand what these three sub-types represent.

1. **Sensory memory** – this category includes memories created through the introduction of ordinary stimuli such as hearing street noises, feeling the warmth of the sun, tasting a sandwich during lunchtime, etc.

Sensory memory is the most temporary form of human memory. For example, if you see a dog while driving to work, chances are you will not remember much about the animal unless you make the conscious effort to remember what you saw.

Sensory memory is active whenever stimulus is present. If you choose to touch the surface of an apple, you will be aware and remember that the apple is smooth. If you decide to smell the apple, you will be aware that in addition to being smooth, the apple also smells very good. Once the stimulus is gone, the sensory memory also disappears.

2. **Short-term memory** – Short-term memory allows people to momentarily remember specific details that they encounter in daily life. Short-term memory works efficiently as long as the individual is actively keeping the detail at the forefront of his thinking.

When a person asks for directions to a nearby town and was told to "go straight, and then take a left at the next road", that person will be able to retain the instructions given because of his short-term memory.

If no active *memory encoding* is performed, most of the details of the conversation with another person will be forgotten.

In a way, short-term memory and sensory memory are similar because they require active, conscious brain use in order to be utilized.

Sensory memory is activated through the five senses, while short-term memory is activated when a person is really thinking about information that he has just received.

3. **Long-term memory** – When a person has to remember information that has to be recalled repeatedly over a period of time, long-term memory is utilized. Imagine the human memory as being structurally composed of three large levels. Each level is filled with an infinite number of information slots.

Two memory levels easily discard information, while the third memory level is dedicated to *keeping* information for long periods of time.

This level is long-term memory. Our focus is to zero in on this memory level and *maximize* its usage and retrieval system. Because who wouldn't want to maximize an organic data bank that has *unlimited capacity*?

The Goal of Memory Improvement

If your goal is to maximize the long-term memory level of the brain, what you really want to do on a more regular basis is to *encode* information *to* this level of the human memory so that we can be more retentive and recall much easier.

Too often, people make the mistake of trusting their short-term memory for *every bit of information* that comes their way. No proper encoding was done, and therefore, the long-term memory is not maximized.

What are the benefits of memory improvement? The answer to this question really depends on your station in life.

For students, improved memory means the active learning process would be much more pleasurable to engage in.

There would be no need to fear any form of examination because your mind has been conditioned to retrieve important information at a moment's notice. Your ability to retain and recall information will also improve long after you have encoded the information in your long-term memory.

For people who are home taking care of their families, improved memory means you won't forget important dates and tasks (such as driving a child to an important school event). Improved memory also means that you will no longer be dependent on physical lists (i.e. "to do" lists, shopping lists, etc.).

For employees, having a more efficient memory translates to better job performance which can positively impact your chances of advancing your career in a company. You will also feel less stressed because you can easily remember all the tasks that have been given to you.

For business people, better memory will allow you to manage every aspect of your business more easily because you remember even the small details.

Some of you may be wondering: how come we can remember specific things while we tend to forget the name of the person who was just introduced to us a few hours ago? The answer lies in the way a person *encodes* the information.

We tend to remember information that has emotions attached to it.

For example, a person who can easily recall the name of his first crush will have difficulty remembering the prices of different fruits in a new grocery store. The difference between these two pieces of information lies in the specific experiences associated with the information.

When a person develops a crush on someone, there is excitement and happiness. Inversely, reading the prices of commodities is about as exciting as watching two old turtles race each other.

So it really doesn't matter *how long* you've had the information, it's how you've encoded the information in your memory. This natural ability to recall very old bits of information is just a normal function of human memory and can be utilized to recall everyday information.

Chapter 3

Human Memory Myths

> *"Each day of our lives we make deposits in the memory banks of our children."*
>
> **Charles R. Swindoll**

There are some general preconceptions about human memory that have to be debunked first before any real memory improvement technique can be put into action.

Myth # 1: Age is the only determining factor that negatively impacts human memory. The more we age, the poorer our memory becomes, and in old age, it is impossible to improve one's memory.

Truly, age affects all organs and organ systems in the body. But when it comes to human memory, healthy individuals must not blame poor recall on age *alone*. Age is just *one* of many factors that affect memory. As people grow older, there is a tendency to blame age for just about anything.

But is age *really* the culprit here? If you can think back to your more youthful years, do you really have *better recall* then than now? Or were you less worried about your memory back then because you had fewer tasks and responsibilities?

Older people are usually more *sensitive* to memory lapses.

And the stress brought about by this super-sensitivity to forgetfulness doesn't help a bit when they are trying to come up with strategies to remedy the forgetfulness. To help evaluate why you are becoming more forgetful, here are some guiding questions:

- Are you more anxious *now* about forgetting things easily?

- How busy are you at work or at home?

- Do you regularly multitask at work?

- Do you have to manage a higher level of stress at this point in time?

- Has your level of physical fitness decreased?

If you have answered 'yes' to some or all of these questions, then your forgetfulness may have been brought about by factors *other* than aging.

Anxiety can easily cause forgetfulness because instead of regularly encoding information in your long-term memory, you are focused on worrying.

Having more responsibilities at work and at school also affects a person's ability to store information for long-term use because people tend to become more selective of what they *want* to remember.

Multitasking, on the other hand, makes full use of short-term memory rather than long-term memory. In the long-term, this affects a person's ability to utilize long-term memory to get through the day's tasks.

The physical health of a person also has a major bearing on a person's memory.

High levels of stress and lack of physical fitness can negatively impact not only your memory, but also your cognitive faculties.

In fact, countless studies in the U.S. and elsewhere point to the increased incidence of dementia and Alzheimer's disease in people who do not regularly exercise and fail to improve their physical fitness in their advanced age.

Myth # 2: If you need to recall something really important, all you have to do is to repeat the information over and over until it is permanently stuck in your long-term memory.

This preconception is based on the belief that the human brain works a bit like our muscles. The more you 'exercise' the brain through mindless memorization, the better.

Unfortunately, there is no proof that plain repetition can help a person improve his memory. Repetition can be used, but it should be part of a larger memory improvement strategy. If used on its own, repetition doesn't really help a person recall anything for the long term.

Myth # 3: The human brain is so powerful that you can train it to never forget things that you want to remember until the end.

The human brain is an amazing organ. The amount of information that you can actively store in it is unlimited – but this doesn't mean that you will be able to remember each every bit of information that you *want* to remember.

It is a given that you will remember many experiences that have had immense significance in your life – but this is about it. Don't expect to remember every face and name that you come across in your lifetime, because human memory just doesn't store information like that.

Myth # 4: Forgetting in itself is a sign of mental weakness and should be avoided at all cost.

Some people think that forgetting is equivalent to weakness. It really isn't because forgetting allows the brain to clear its memory of unnecessary clutter.

If the human memory *never forgets* anything, people would have difficulty sorting through all the information stored in the long-term memory.

What we want to develop is a strong recall system for *important information* only. But for unimportant input, you can forget those things without feeling guilty or weak.

Myth # 5: The best possible way to improve one's memory is to use visualization techniques.

Many memory improvement strategies make use of visualization to help people remember the most mundane things (like shopping lists).

While visualizing concepts and words can help to a certain extent, one should note that visualization is not the *only* way to improve one's memory.

For example, visualization doesn't help a person remember long strings of numbers or complicated physics formulas, though it can help someone remember diagrams.

It really depends on *what you need to accomplish*. The memory improvement strategy should always be congruent with what you want to encode and recall.

Chapter 4

Memory Busters

> *"A lot of people mistake a short memory for a clear conscience".*
>
> **Doug Larson**

Are you puzzled by the sudden inability to recall information? Check out our list of three common memory busters and see if one or all of these factors are negatively affecting your own memory.

Memory Buster # 1: Stress

Stress is very common in modern society. It affects not only our physical health but also our mental well-being.

In addition to reducing a person's focus and mental stamina, recent studies show that people who are unable to effectively manage stress have a higher risk for memory problems than people who know how to de-stress regularly.

It turns out that stress has a *biological effect* on human memory.

If a person is always stressed, the brain cells in the learning region of the human brain have a hard time communicating with each other. If brain cells are unable to communicate effectively, retention and recall will be affected greatly since human memory is very dependent on these nerve processes.

Too much stress also takes away much needed glucose and oxygen *away* from the brain.

The body produces two kinds of hormones that allow a person to engage in fight-or-flight behavior: cortisol and adrenaline. Under normal circumstances, the presence of these hormones can definitely help a person save himself from dangerous situations (e.g. physical attacks from other people, emergency situations, etc.).

But here's what happens when a person *continues* to feel stressed (say, for an entire day, or even for *weeks*): the body will cease producing adrenaline (the primary fight-or-flight hormone) and will start producing large amounts of cortisol.

Cortisol diverts sugar and oxygen from the brain and other organs, and this reduces the total energy that the brain can use for its vital functions. With less energy to use, the brain's processes suffer. If a person is under stress for more than three days, memory problems begin to emerge.

Now, there is no need to feel even more stressed by this news because if you can *reduce* the amount of stress in your life through stress management techniques like massage, recreation, hypnosis, or autogenic techniques, your memory will revert to its normal state within just *seven days*.

Memory Buster # 2: Sleep

For many of us, not having enough sleep is just a fact of life. We all have 'sleep debts' that we try to pay off with extra snoozing whenever we have some free time for rest. Sadly, only a small fraction of people with large sleep debts *ever* recover from having too little sleep.

So how does chronic lack of sleep affect people? Here are some of the more common effects:

- Frequent tension headaches

- Individuals with migraine headaches suffer from more frequent attacks

- There is also an emotional impact (e.g. people are easily angered or saddened)

- Focus is reduced

- Drive to finish projects and tasks are reduced

- Forgetfulness / temporary memory impairment

According to new studies, a person who says he feels quite rested after only a few hours of sleep will not be able to outperform a person who has had almost eight hours of sleep. This applies to people who sleep less than seven hours on most days.

If your work involves a lot of mental work, it would do well for you to sleep *at least* seven hours every night. It has been found that going without sleep for a full twenty-four hours can make a person behave as if he had drank four full glasses of wine, one after another!

So how much sleep does the average individual need? The following list will help shed some light on this:

Age	Average Number of Hours of Sleep Needed Every Night
29 days – 12 months	16 hours
1 – 3 years	11 hours
3 – 6 years	11 hours
6 – 12 years	10 hours
12 – 19 years	9 hours
19 years and above	8 – 9 hours

If you are known to sleep less than seven hours every day, it is time to change your sleeping patterns, because not only is your memory impaired by a chronic lack of sleep, but research has also shown that people who sleep *less* than the recommended "sleep allowance" for adults have a higher mortality rate.

If you are enjoying your golden years, there is no reason to sleep fewer hours per day. Sure, you may be sleeping more lightly now, but you still need an average of eight hours of sleep every night. Do it for better health – and better memory.

Need another reason to start sleeping longer, every night? Here it is: the brain needs sleep to consolidate new information. Memory consolidation or the storage of information to long-term memory *only occurs* when a person is sleeping. Here's how it works:

1. New information is encoded through stimuli.

2. Person actively encodes the new information.

3. Information is *temporarily* placed in the hippocampus.

4. Person goes to sleep.

5. Brain waves transfer the information from the hippocampus to another region of the brain (the neocortex).

Some people might be asking: is it enough to take naps if regular sleep at night is not possible? Unfortunately, no. You need regular sleep before this transfer process can take place. Don't forget that the quality of your sleep every night also has a bearing on memory consolidation, so take the steps to correct any sleep problems you may have presently.

Memory Buster # 3: Multitasking

Multitasking may well be the hallmark of modern living. Many people find it *impossible* to get through an entire day without doing two or three things at once.

While it is true that multitasking somewhat improves a person's productivity (especially in a hectic office setting), did you know that this practice has a negative effect on the human memory?

According to recent studies, people who multitask don't actually focus on two or three things *at once*.

It may appear that a person is doing so many things at one time, but according to brain scans performed by U.S. researchers, the human brain can actually focus on just *one* task at a time. The brain 'switches' from one task to another instead of simultaneously performing two tasks at the same time.

So how does this affect a person's memory? When the human brain tries to encode information while a person is multitasking, the brain actually tries to record information from *both* activities.

This parallel information processing causes recall problems because a person may not be able to recall the information from *one* activity without recalling the information from the *other* activity.

For example, if a person was listening to a colleague while watching a video message, he may not be able to fully remember what the colleague was saying if he does not try to remember what he was watching *while* he was listening to another person.

Is there a way to improve your memory while multitasking? Not really, because improving one's memory also has a lot to do with increasing one's *focus*.

You either focus a hundred percent on *one activity* or you split your attention to accomplish two activities. So for your memory's sake, it would be better if you avoided multitasking altogether so you can focus *and retain* information better.

Chapter 5

Boosting Memory From Within

> *"Many a man fails as an original thinker simply because his memory is too good."*
>
> **Friedrich Nietzsche**

So far we have been able to explore the various factors that may have an adverse effect on a person's memory. We have discovered that a person with declining memory can be affected by a myriad of factors, not just aging.

Now, to truly improve one's memory, we should adopt a *holistic* strategy that acknowledges the importance of the *mind-body connection*.

What does this mean? If the body is healthy, it follows that you will be more mentally fit than those who ignore their own physical health. There are some steps that you can take to ensure that you are doing *everything you can* to maintain a healthy brain.

The Cholesterol-Memory Connection

Recent studies have shown that people with high levels of LDL or bad cholesterol have a higher risk of cognitive decline in advanced age.

Such individuals also have a higher risk of developing debilitating conditions like Alzheimer's disease. Cognitive decline has a negative impact on a person's ability to retain and recall information and also makes learning much more difficult.

Individuals with high cholesterol levels are usually unaware of their condition because high LDL levels in the bloodstream usually do not produce any discomfort.

People who have never consulted with their physicians regarding their cholesterol level usually find out too late that their LDL levels have spiraled. High cholesterol levels, as you may already know, also predispose a person to stroke and heart attacks.

It is possible to reverse high cholesterol by modifying one's diet and by engaging in light to moderate exercise (at least thirty minutes every day). In some cases, a person may be prescribed *statins*.

There is no need to avoid taking medication for cholesterol because statins have been proven to *lower the risk* for Alzheimer's disease. So you are actually shooting two birds with one stone by following your doctor's recommendation. Here are some more ways to take charge of high cholesterol levels:

1. The average cholesterol requirement of adults is only 300 milligrams *per day*. To maintain low LDL levels, it is recommended that you look closely at the nutritional labels of commercially sold food items. The lower your cholesterol intake per day, the better.

2. The body can dispose of excess cholesterol through the digestive tract – it only needs *one thing* to accomplish this: *dietary fiber*. If you cannot get enough fiber from your daily diet, consider investing in fiber supplements to help improve your digestion, and at the same time, help your body get rid of excess cholesterol.

3. Omega-3 fatty acids help combat the negative effects of high cholesterol in the body. Fish is a natural source of omega-3. To

get enough omega-3, consider replacing most of the meat in your diet with cold-water fishes.

4. Smoking causes bodily inflammation and magnifies the deleterious effects of high cholesterol. Reduce your cigarette consumption or quit the habit altogether.

5. There are two types of cholesterol in the body – high-density lipoproteins and low-density lipoproteins. The former is classified as "good cholesterol" while the latter is the "bad cholesterol" that is often the target of anti-cholesterol medication like statins.

   If you dislike the idea of taking statins in the future, you have to start exercising more *now* because adequate physical activity actually *reduces* the amount of low-density lipoproteins in the body and maintains the level of good cholesterol.

6. Excessive alcohol intake is bad for both the heart and your memory. If you have the habit of consuming more than two glasses of liquor every night, you are *not* helping improve your cholesterol profile.

Reduce your intake and switch to *red wine*. Red wine is full of the super-antioxidant *resveratrol*, which has been noted for its ability to reduce bad cholesterol.

Memory Impairment & Homocysteine

Homocysteine is a building block of protein structures in the human body. The body naturally produces it and allows it to flow freely in the bloodstream.

Whenever protein structures have to be created, homocysteine is transformed with the help of vitamin B12. Here's the problem – not everyone has adequate vitamin B12 in their diets. However, we should note that diet is not the sole culprit when it comes to vitamin B12 deficiency.

There are some instances when a person has an autoimmune condition that prevents the body from absorbing and using the vital vitamin. The result is that the body continues to produce homocysteine and it *accumulates*.

What does this have to do with your memory? Well, current research has shown that people with high levels of homocysteine also have a higher risk of developing Alzheimer's disease in advanced age. It has also been discovered that plaque formation in brain tissue increases over time if high homocysteine levels are not regulated.

Chapter 6

How Diet Can Help Your Brain

> *"Memory... is the diary that we all carry about with us."*
> **Oscar Wilde**

Diet plays a vital role in creating balance in the human body and also prevents damage to the brain from oxidative stress.

A diet rich in natural antioxidants can help reduce inflammation and free radical damage to *all* of the body's various organs, including the brain. Simply put: if you have an antioxidant rich diet, your brain and memory will function better - even in old age.

Controlled studies in the United States have pointed to the following food items as being rich in natural antioxidants:

- *Spinach*
- *Curcumin*
- *Blueberries*
- *Walnuts*
- *Pecans*
- *Cherries*
- *Green tea*
- *Broccoli*

Of course, you still have to watch your sugar and salt intake when integrating these items into your daily diet so you that you'll be able to reap the full benefits without raising your blood glucose level or sodium intake.

If you have had a high-fat diet for many, many years, then chances are there is a lot of inflammation resulting from a lack of specific vitamins.

You can try vitamin supplementation to reduce tissue inflammation in your body and to protect your brain. The following vitamins are a good choice because these vitamins have been known to disable free radicals and protect the nervous system as well:

- *Vitamin E*
- *Vitamin D*

- *Vitamin C*
- *Vitamin B12*

All these vitamins can be sourced from health supplements and from fresh fruits and vegetables.

You can also get vitamin D by exposing yourself daily to a healthy amount of natural sunlight – your body will naturally produce the vitamin for you.

Vitamin D is an extra important vitamin because research shows that individuals whose cognitive function have declined steadily over a period of years have low levels of free vitamin D in their bloodstream.

Folate, on the other hand, is another important nutrient that protects the brain and nervous system – you should also get *sufficient amounts* of this nutrient by eating enriched breads and by increasing your intake of fresh vegetables.

Dietary sources of cobalamin or vitamin B12 include:

- *Dairy products* (choose enriched, low-fat dairy products)

- *Lean meat* (avoid red meat as this increases bad *cholesterol*)
- *Poultry* (trim the fat from the meat and remove the skin)
- *Cold water fish*
- *Seafood*

Dietary sources of folate include:

- *Leafy veggies*
- *White beans*
- *Red beans*
- *Beet*
- *Fresh tomatoes & tomato products*
- *Citrus fruits*
- *Soy products*

You can get tocopherol or naturally occurring vitamin E from:
- *Vegetable oil*
- *Leafy veggies*
- *Root crops*
- *Avocado*

Additional Guidelines to Boost Your Memory

1. Check your sight and hearing – minor vision loss and impaired hearing can also affect a person's memory.

Sharper senses lead to better information encoding and recall. Always remember that a person's ability to recall is drastically affected by the efficiency at which a person is able to receive sensory input.

2. Do you have maintenance medication for any health condition? If you do, you may want to check the side effects of the prescription drugs that you are taking on a daily basis.

If the medical literature states that you may feel slight grogginess or memory impairment, you have the option of consulting with your physician for an alternative prescription if you think your medication is interfering with your ability to remember even the most common things.

3. In addition to getting enough sleep at night, a person must also manage fatigue efficiently to improve his memory. Fatigue is caused by a myriad of factors, not just physical activity or long working hours.

For example, excessive coffee consumption or increased sugar intake can also exacerbate the symptoms of fatigue in the long-term because the body becomes dependent on short bursts of energy.

A Fit Body Creates a Fit Mind & Memory

As we have mentioned earlier in the book, physical fitness plays a role in maintaining a healthy mind. This, in turn, creates an efficient memory that will serve a person for decades to come.

But the main problem with today's fast-paced lifestyle is that it does not allow a person to set aside some time for regular exercise. If you are encountering the same problems, here are some tips to get you started:

1. Some people put exercise in their "least priority" list. It's time to reverse this harmful trend. Instead of putting off exercise, make it the *number one priority* every day. And you don't have to exercise for half an hour in the beginning.

    If you can devote just fifteen minutes of your time to light to moderate exercise (such as jogging or walking), you can gradually increase the duration of your exercise as you go along.

    This way, your mind and body will be able to adapt to your new activity. Eventually, exercise will become part of your daily routine and you will feel that your day isn't complete without exercise.

2. Never attempt to start an exercise regimen with high-impact exercises lasting for more than one hour every day. You will exhaust yourself (and tire your muscles) so much that you will probably quit in one week and never try again.

3. Physical fitness is more effective if you set goals for yourself – so you can reward yourself in the end when these goals are achieved. But be careful when setting goals for yourself – unrealistic goals can drain your motivation and enthusiasm.

4. If walking, jogging and curl ups don't sound enjoyable to you (and people rarely find these exercises enjoyable), the best way to start a new physical fitness regimen is by finding a sport that you like.

Who knows? Maybe you have a killer basketball shot or you are really a tennis ace in the making. Try different sports and settle for a sport that you would *love* to engage in month after month.

Increasing your physical activity should not be limited to weekend visits to the gym or daily exercise. You have to increase your physical activity throughout the day to ensure that you are burning more excess calories *effortlessly*.

You can do this by parking your vehicle farther from your office building (so you can walk the rest of the way), avoiding elevators/lifts, and walking to nearby locations instead of driving there.

A ten to fifteen-minute walk is reasonable – and you might be surprised at the distance you can reach with just fifteen minutes of walking.

5. We are all familiar with events that involve "running for a cause" or "walking for a cause".

   Instead of ignoring invitations to such events, why not join one? It won't hurt to support a cause you like and you would be meeting new people while getting the exercise you need!

6. Your coworkers probably need motivation to exercise, too. It won't hurt to ask your closest office mates if they want to join you in your

sport (and vice versa). A 'fitness team' can be formed.

7. You also have to remind yourself *why* you are doing this in the first place. You want to live longer. You don't want to suffer from heart disease, heart attacks and stroke. You want to see your kids grow up to have kids of their own. Your personal motivation should be at the very center of the fitness effort.

Socializing With Others Matters

Believe it or not, having a good social life also affects your memory's capacity to function efficiently as you age.

It has been proven that people who always stay at home and make the conscious effort to avoid speaking and socialize with other people are more prone to memory impairment and cognitive decline than folks who go out of their way to strengthen bonds with existing friends and make an effort to find new ones.

If you are not interested in finding people that you can invite to dinner, that's no problem. What people really need is to *reach out* and socialize with others. A good start would be to find an organization or club that interests you.

Whether you are into beekeeping or photography, we are quite certain that there is an organization out there made up of like-minded individuals that can cater to your needs. By socializing with people more, you can cut your risk for degenerative mental conditions by as much as fifty percent.

Chapter 7

Memory Solutions

> *"There are lots of people who mistake their imagination for their memory."*
>
> **Josh Billings**

Kinds of Memory Loss

There are two main types of memory loss: early memory loss and advanced memory loss. Early memory loss is usually normal and is not regularly associated with diseases such as Alzheimer's.

Advanced memory loss, on the other hand, may be a sign that a person is suffering from a more severe condition. In such cases, consult with your physician immediately.

Early Memory Loss

Early memory loss usually involves:

- Inability to find the *right word* for a particular expression

- Inability to recall a person after his or her name has been said

- Forgetting where you placed small items like keys, rings and watches

- Inability to recall what specific day it is

- Forgetting some items from a list of things to do

- Missing one or two appointments

- Disorientation in large spaces like shopping malls

Advanced Memory Loss

The following are signs of advanced memory loss:

- Inability to name day-to-day items like tables, chairs, identification cards, etc.

- The person finds it difficult to communicate because he/she is unable to understand common words.

- Word substitution becomes more frequent, to the point that the person's speech becomes incomprehensible or unintelligible.

- People with advanced memory loss also tend to ask questions repeatedly, even if an appropriate answer or response has already been given.

- Associations become more muddled. A person with advanced memory loss may accidentally place an item (like a hammer) and place it in an inappropriate location (e.g. a freezer). It is common for such individuals to forget how such items were placed in strange locations.

- Forgetting what month or year it is.

- Inappropriate clothing choice is also a sign of advanced memory loss.

For example, a person with advanced memory loss may choose to wear loose summer clothes during the wintertime and not be aware of the discrepancy between the time of the year and the clothing choice.

- Moving around in one's neighborhood becomes difficult; the person may get lost even if he has lived in that particular neighborhood for years.

- Inability to recall why you are in a certain place or forgetting how you arrived in that location in the first place

Chapter 8

Sharpening Your Five Senses

> *"So long as the memory of certain beloved friends lives in my heart, I shall say that life is good."*
>
> **Helen Keller**

As we have discussed earlier, the five senses have a direct bearing on a person's memory.

So if you want to improve your memory, you have to sharpen your senses. The following exercise will serve to challenge the way you store and recall information collected through the various senses.

Exercise # 1: The Eyes

Materials:
Pen
Paper

Medium-sized picture
Stopwatch

The exercise:

1. Find a quiet spot in your home and take a seat. When you are ready, take a look at the medium-sized picture for just 30 seconds. Use the stopwatch to monitor your viewing time.

2. After the 30 seconds have passed, quickly place the picture face down on the table (no peeking!)

3. List as many details as you can about the picture that you have just viewed. There is no time limit for this part of the exercise. Take as long as you want in listing the unique details.

4. When you are done listing the details, get the picture and compare the details that you have listed and the actual details that you were *referring to* in the picture. Are there any discrepancies? Note the discrepancies and note the details that you were not able to list.

5. Try to figure out why you were not able to recall other details about the picture.

Repeat this simple sight exercise every day to increase your mind's ability to keep track of even the smallest visual details. Also, never forget to perform an evaluation after every exercise to track your progress.

Exercise # 2: The Ears

Materials:

Music player
Pen
Paper
Audio recorder

The exercise:

Hearing is often considered inferior to sight (since many people are more visual than auditory) – but this does not mean that hearing doesn't provide the same level of stimulation or *input* as sight. The following exercises will focus on 'teasing' your sense of hearing so you can be as receptive to sound *as much* as you are to visual input.

Exercise 2.1

Pick your favorite song and listen to it carefully with your music player. Now get a pen and some paper and write down *everything you can* about the song.

Note the music flow, the tone of the singer's voice, etc. If you don't want to write down the details, you can just record your observations using an audio recorder.

Play the music again and compare the details that you have just written or recorded with the actual musical piece. Now, play the music again from the very start and record details about the music *as the music is playing*. Compare the music and your notes once again.

Exercise 2.2

Watch a DVD movie on your computer or on your home entertainment system. Now close your eyes and try to imagine what is happening in the TV show or movie by just using your sense of hearing.

For this exercise, you will need an audio recorder because you will have to record what you think is happening in the movie *visually* as you listen to the sounds and dialog.

After 10 to 15 minutes, stop recording and compare your audio notes with what is actually happening in the movie. How accurate was your recreation of the visual scenes while your eyes were closed?

Exercise 2.3

If you are the type of person who usually says "can you say that again?" your problem is probably not your memory but your inability to engage in *active listening*. Active listening involves concentrating on the input of the person you are speaking to *instead* of formulating responses as bits of information come in.

Remember our earlier discussion about multitasking? The brain is unable to focus on two things at once. So when you are speaking to someone, it would be better if you gave a hundred percent attention to the other person through active listening, instead of splitting your attention every time you speak to someone.

You can try active listening anywhere – at home, at church, at work or even when you are at the gym. All you have to do is to completely suspend the urge to shoot back a response and just *listen deeply* to what the other person is saying *before* formulating a reply.

Exercise 2.4

Assuming that you have normal hearing (if the opposite is true, you can skip this exercise), it's now time to see how observant you can be by just using your sense of hearing.

Sit in a very quiet part of the house (no kids, no pets, no ringing phones, etc.) Take a few minutes to get accustomed to the silence of the environment. Close your eyes and take note of *everything* that you can hear from the quiet room. You might be surprised at how many sounds there are.

Exercise # 3: The Skin

Materials:

Assorted small items like children's toys & household items
Handkerchief

The exercise:

The skin has been blessed by Mother Nature with millions of sensitive nerve cells that convey even the slightest changes in pressure. This allows human beings to survive in so many different conditions.

You may not be aware of it, but one's sense of touch is just as powerful as the other senses and it also helps us create vivid memories of situations and individual experiences.

It will be much better if someone else can prepare the small items for you. That way, you will be completely unaware of what is in front of you. If you are ready, take a seat behind a small table and put on the blindfold (the handkerchief).

Tell your companion to place all the items on the table. Pick up each of the items and try to tell what it was just by feeling each item with your hands. Take note of the physical characteristics of each of the items and try to attach a particular emotion to each physical sensation.

When you are done, take off the blindfold and write down the details that you have just created in your mind on a piece of paper. Repeat this exercise as many times as you like – the more you try this exercise, the more open your mind will be to informational input from your sense of touch.

Exercise # 4: The Tongue

Materials:

An assortment of food items
Pen
Paper
Audio recorder
Handkerchief

The exercise:

Have you ever heard of professional tasters and professional smellers? Perfume companies and companies from the food and beverage industries hire these folks to make sure that their products will be successful in whatever market they belong to.

Professional tasters specifically, have been trained to recall *thousands* of different tastes and scents (because you won't be able to taste anything if you can't smell anything).

These individuals are called organoleptic because they have trained specific senses to pick up on details that ordinary individuals cannot. For instance, an organoleptic would be able to say if a particular batch of coffee was too oily or too fruity.

An interesting fact about organoleptic people is that they have not been blessed with any special abilities, other than their determination to succeed as professional tasters and smellers.

These folks do not have extra large noses or extra sensitive tongues. What they do have is an immense receptivity to sensory input – something that has naturally increased their memory power over the years.

You can achieve the same results by doing this particular exercise. Now, to facilitate the tasting of the assortment of foods that have been prepared, you will need another person to give you each food, one after the other. Put on the blindfold before the food is brought to you.

You have two choices: you can either taste the food first then record your input later, or you can record your observations as you taste the food, one by one. Focus on the texture and the various tastes that every bit of the food has.

Exercise # 5: The Nose

Materials:

Audio recorder
Pen
Paper
Small food items, household items, items found outside your home (e.g. leaves, flowers, etc.)

The exercise:

This exercise is similar to the earlier exercise; the only difference is that you will be using your sense of smell. You still have to record your observations on paper after the exercise.

Chapter 9

Brain Workouts

> *"I have a writer's memory which makes everything worse than maybe it actually was."*
>
> **Amy Tan**

Believe it or not, the brain needs to be exercised in order to be in top condition. Brain exercise is essentially a creative stimulation of the gray matter. The following are some ways that you can exercise your brain to improve information recall and other brain functions:

Activities that force you to think continually from start to finish:

- Assembling a model train or model car

- Trying to answer questions from a tough TV quiz program

- Designing a new culinary masterpiece in your own kitchen (without the help of existing recipes)

- Answering Sudoku puzzles, "word find" games, and crosswords

Activities that break existing routines:

- Trying to find an alternate route to your office building, even if it means getting lost a bit

- If you are a right-handed person, try brushing with your left hand (and vice versa)

- Assuming that you regularly eat with Western utensils, try eating your entire dinner with a pair of chopsticks

Activities that challenge your ability to learn something completely new:

- Assuming that you are a native English speaker, try learning Chinese or French

- Don't have any hobbies right now? It's time to find a new passion.

- Never made a functioning website in your life? Try making one in the next few days – from scratch.

- Learn to play the violin, drums, guitar or xylophone. Pick a musical instrument that you like and start learning how to play it.

Activities that introduce different modes of thought:

- Write a 10-stanza poem with rhyming endings

- Get a large block of ice and try to create art through ice sculpting

- Sketch anything using regular watercolor, charcoal, pencil or even pastel

- Your autobiography won't write itself – why not try starting today?

- Love romance novels? Try reading action-adventure novels for a change.

General Guidelines for Efficient Recall

Memory improvement requires a certain discipline that can be achieved through the practice of certain general principles.

The following general principles can be applied to just about any memory improvement technique. Use these guidelines to enhance your current knowledge and practice of active memory improvement.

1. Meaningful associations of concepts or words will always be easier to recall. So whenever you are creating associations, always keep in mind your personality and *what matters to you* to help create images that can be easily recalled at a moment's notice.

2. It is possible to organize or group information in your memory. You just have to focus on creating appropriate hierarchies to make information easier to retrieve at a later time.

   If you like organizing physical documents, use the same techniques you use to file away important information. Use visual techniques to master these new hierarchies that you have created to enhance your long-term memory.

3. There are two groups of learners: those who like to think in pictures (visual learners) and those who prefer hearing and rehearsing words (auditory learners). Always choose a memory improvement technique that fits your own personal way of learning to accelerate your progress and minimize failure.

4. Use all your senses when attempting to store new information. We have devoted an entire chapter of this book to sharpening all five senses.

5. If a series of mnemonic images don't make sense when you just imagine them visually, try creating rhymes to help your memory store the new information.

6. Large tracts of information are easier to remember if you are able to separate the information into discernable chunks.

7. Always pay close attention to whatever is happening in front of you, because the human brain can only process about 10% of all the sensory input you have at any given time.

8. When there is no conscious effort to remember new information, the information will most likely be encoded into short-term memory and will be forgotten within the day.

9. Attempting to transfer information from short-term memory to long-term memory will be difficult if you usually multitask for most of the day.

10. Memorization requires at least three attempts before information can be successfully transferred to long-term memory.

11. Rehearsing information (or memorization) can be effective if you introduce variations to the material as you go along. Simply put, if you can make things interesting, you brain will find it easier to remember things.

Chapter 10

Memory Improvement Strategies

> *"One ought to have a good memory when he has told a lie."*
>
> Pierre Corneille

The following are memory improvement techniques that can be used for a variety of circumstances. Try one, several or all of these strategies and see which one works for your needs.

Strategy # 1: The Power of Mnemonics

Mnemonics is a memory improvement technique that makes full use of *associations* to improve retention and recall of particular bits of information.

The system was developed by the ancient Greeks (the term "mnemonics" was derived from Mnemosyne, a Greek deity) who discovered early on that human memory thrived with associative operations.

A good example of this would be when we think of ordinary objects. Think of any fruit right now. Once you actively think of a particular fruit, your memory retrieves not only the name and *meaning* of the name, but also brings to the forefront the *various characteristics* of the fruit.

If you thought of an apple, you could probably shoot a chain of descriptive words right away: red, shiny, crisp, sweet, tasty, etc. Your memory was able to recall such an impressive group of concepts and words because you have actively associated bits of information with each other.

This is not the limit of concept association – because you can actually take associations *further* to create specialized memories that would allow you to recall longer and more difficult bits of information. To summarize, you can use associations to recall *anything* that you want to remember later on.

Mnemonics can be achieved by making use of the three core concepts behind it:

1. Associating images, concepts and information

2. Imagining or animating the associated concepts in your mind

3. Contextualizing and differentiating mnemonic systems through location

The first concept, active association of information, is the *most important* guiding principle behind mnemonics. Without association, you would have nothing to actively imagine, encode and recall in the first place. Association is considered the base or foundation of any mnemonic system.

So how is association achieved? Association is achieved when new information (e.g. information that has to be recalled at a later time) is combined or associated with pre-existing information in your memory. To clarify further: the first bit of information is new/foreign at the moment while the second bit of information is old/familiar.

You have probably used a mnemonic device in the past to remember tough lessons at school; you just weren't familiar with the formal technique.

See? This memory improvement technique is fairly ordinary. What we're doing is simply furthering the technique that you have been using for a long time so you can start strategically creating your own mnemonic systems when you have to remember something.

Some people think that the only way that you can associate concepts is by creating a rational series of concepts or words.

The association is often expressed as phrases or concepts. While this approach to creating a mnemonic system is completely acceptable, one should note that you can be more creative with your associations.

Here are some examples of creative, non-conventional associations (note the bolded terms):

1. The yellow bird is **on top** of the green alien.

2. Number 8 **crashed** into number 2, while number 3 was **absorbed** by number 7.

3. The bear and the washing machine **merged** to become a cleaning robot.

4. The table **wrapped around** the golden dollar sign.

5. Numbers 9, 5, 6 and 7 are **dancing around** a campfire.

6. The fish, oven toaster and modem are **all colored** red

These are just a few of the ways that you can visually combine two unlike concepts. Associations do not have to be rational at all. In fact, for the purpose of quicker recall, the funnier and more absurd the connection between two unlike concepts, the better off you would be.

Now, where do the two other concepts (imagining and location) fall into the scheme of things? We can consider these two other concepts as *passive processes* that take place as one tries to recall an association. Imagination is the way you recall the association so you can trigger the recall of the actual information.

The tone, mood and emotions of the association become animate during the imagining phase. As for location, you would only need to use this if you have similar mnemonic systems that you would have to use all at once (e.g. an examination where there are intersecting concepts and theories).

For example, you can set one mnemonic system in the North Pole (this is just a striking, visual location that would allow you to differentiate a chain of associations), while the second mnemonic system is set in a hot beach.

See the contrast? The differences will allow you to carefully recall all the concepts that you set out to remember without mixing or confusing associations with each other.

Here's a quick exercise: let's say you want to remember a group of words *in a particular order*.

1. Mouse
2. Banana
3. Hat
4. Light bulb
5. Scissors
6. Table
7. Grapes
8. Conductor
9. Car
10. Snake

The last paragraph contains a list of words that you should try to remember using a mnemonic system. We will be providing examples or 'mnemonic images' below, but you should create your own system, too.

1. A mouse is being ridden by a gigantic, yellow banana.
2. A pink hat is worn by a laughing, yellow light bulb.
3. A pair of scissors is wrestling with a scratched table.
4. A stout conductor is eating a bowl of grapes.
5. 5. A car is racing with a speedy snake.

If you imagined the mnemonic images we have just given you, you should be able to recall *all* the items on the list *in that particular order*. So as you can see, mnemonics actually reduces the amount of information that you have to directly commit to memory by substituting text and concepts with images.

Tips for Better Mnemonics

While you are free to experiment with mnemonics to help you in your day-to-day problems with remembering things, here are some tips you can follow to improve your success rate:

1. You are encouraged to be as creative as you can with your associations, however, you should avoid visually negative or violent

associations (e.g. a cobra trying to kill a rattlesnake) because these associations are actually *more difficult to recall* in a series. Stick to positive associations (or at least, neutral associations) so you can recall the mnemonic images quickly.

2. Since mnemonics is a *visual* technique, make your mnemonic images as memorable as possible. You can do this easily by exaggerating individual elements of a mnemonic image.

3. Never underestimate the power of humor. The funnier a mnemonic image, the better.

4. Do you need to remember difficult lessons (e.g. the names of towns and cities)? Try rhyming the names and titles.

5. A chain of interrelated concepts can be remembered more easily if you can use shapes *within* the mnemonic device (a mnemonic device doesn't have to be a sentence).

Strategy # 2: Improved Recall Techniques

If you are already in your golden years, recall may be slowly becoming more and more difficult.

There is no need to fret however because there are *three easy ways* that you can improve your recall.

I. Relax before you recall

People often feel anxious (or even scared) when faced with the prospect of recalling old information in front of people (such as recalling the name of a friend back in high school).

This is the most counter-productive way of doing things, because *any form of anxiety* or fear causes 'emotional flooding' which prevents the brain from retrieving information from long-term memory.

So whenever you need to recall something right then and there, you need to calm your nerves to allow your brain to remember the information that you need.

Often, calming yourself can be as easy as relaxing your facial muscles and closing your eyes for a few seconds. Focus on the information retrieval and *not* on your fear of not being able to remember.

There might also be many situations when your brain becomes focused on a particular letter or number.

Never ignore these memory clues, because these clues are also part of the information retrieval process. Learn to trust these small fragments of recall and *keep your mind clear* when you are trying to remember something. If your surrounding area is noisy, block out the noise during the recall.

II. Scour your memory bank

As we have discussed earlier, the brain works well with associations. Individual bits of information can be recalled if you can summon *related information* as you are performing the conscious effort of remembering something. It's easy to scour your memory bank this way if you work with *categories*.

For example, if you are *desperate* to remember a particular film you watched ten years ago, don't waste your efforts by focusing on the content of the movie.

Instead, pan your attention to the various elements *surrounding* the creation of the movie. Try to remember the other movies that were released alongside the film. You can also try to recall movies done by the same actor or actress.

Here are some other ways that you can associate or relate particular information with similar information to help jog your long-term memory.

Technique	Rationale
Going from letters A – Z	It is possible to recall the name of a person, movie or place by getting the first letter of the name correctly. By reciting the letters of the alphabet, there is a chance that you will be able to capture the *first letter* of the word that you are trying to remember.
Revisit the scene	Remembering is also an act of reconstruction because the mind is continually trying to reconstruct the time, place and circumstances where you learned a particular piece of

	information.
	So if you are at a loss when trying to remember something that someone told you in the past, try to imagine the *time and place* when you received the information.
Sensory association	If you were listening to the radio when you received the information that you are now trying to recall, why not try listening to the radio again? By rebuilding the context of the information, your memory would be able to recall more easily.
Counting the steps	Losing your keys, cellular phone or even wallet can be extremely

	frustrating.
	Long-term disorganization can compound this problem; so the best way to recall in such circumstances is by carefully recreating all the steps that you took before reaching a particular point.
	So if you've lost an item, try to think what you were doing within the last half hour before you lost it. Then ask yourself: what was the last thing I did before I lost the item?
Single-event recall	Don't have the time to recall all the stuff that you did prior to coming upon the information or losing that item? Just try to remember what you were doing *at the*

	exact moment.
Printed word recall	Having trouble remembering stuff that you have read in the past? It might help if you recalled what the book or document looked like. Next, try to remember on what particular area or region you read the piece of information.

III. Review

Going to reunions can be tough on someone with some memory loss. Don't be too hard on yourself if you think you won't be able to remember everyone who greets you at the reunion. Revisit school yearbooks so you will be able to review the faces and names of people.

Chapter 11

Beating Absentmindedness

> *"Memory is deceptive because it is colored by today's events."*
>
> **Albert Einstein**

Stress and fatigue can take a toll on a person's memory. If these negative states are not managed properly, your memory and attention can both take a beating; the result would be sheer absentmindedness – and we all know how inconvenient absentmindedness can be.

If you want to conquer absentmindedness, follow these easy steps:

1. Boring routines can exacerbate absentmindedness. Because you don't have to pay attention to things as much because of established routines, you often end up doing

things mechanically, paying no heed to details.

Time to break this cycle. Rock the roof – do things differently. If you usually placed your daily mail on the table, place it somewhere quite unusual – like on outdoor furniture.

2. Small items like keys can get lost easily. If your days are too hectic and stressful, you need just *one place* for all these loose items. A box or a small plastic case would be a great place to drop all those things. That way, your stuff will never get lost.

3. Nearly every new cellular phone model has a "to do" application and calendar/appointment application. Use these programs to remember chores and appointments. Setting alarms at specific hours is a good way to ensure that you never forget important appointments.

4. For those who don't like punching away at their cellular phones all day just to remember things, a small notepad might be a better choice.

A small notepad or notebook that fits in your pocket can serve as the extension of your short-term memory. Just make sure that you scribble *legibly* in your own notebook so you are able to decipher your notes at the end of the day.

5. Your environment can also be used to improve your recall of important things. If you have to visit the dentist at 10 o'clock, you can wear your watch backwards.

    The unusual appearance of your watch will trigger an instant recall of the last important bit of information on your mind. You can do this with other items in your office or house as well. All you need is something *unusual* to remind you of something you need to remember.

6. Though this practice should not be overused, it might help if you write notes to yourself and stuck them on highly visible spots.

7. Multitasking never helps people remember important dates and appointments.

If all else fails, ask someone close to you to remind you of an important event, appointment or chore on the exact day. A call or text message will do.

Pegging Together Ideas

The pegging method of memory improvement makes use of visualization and mnemonic techniques with a twist – it allows you to memorize a series of words and numbers *in order* by creating a continuous chain of memory cues.

Let's take numbers 1 – 10 for example. All you have to do is assign a word to each of the numbers in the series to make each digit more memorable. Rhyming is recommended to make recall easier:

    1 = pun
    2 = boo
    3 = me
    4 = pour
    5 = jibe
    6 = nicks
    7 = raven
    8 = mate
    9 = pine
    10 = hen

That wasn't too difficult, now was it? Now on to step two of the pegging method: you now have to create a memorable series of memory cues with the associations that you have just made. Let's assume that for this particular exercise, you need to remember all the numbers that we have just used *in order:*

> *He made a bad* **pun** *that made the ghost say* **boo. Me** *I like to* **pour** *while I* **jibe** *with my friends. You can get bad* **nicks** *from a wild* **raven** *that wants to* **mate** *while the* **pine** *tree made the* **hen** *feel small.*

As you can see from our example, the memory cues don't have to make any logical sense – but the cues have to be fashioned in such a way that they become even more memorable to you. This feature of memory cues is very important to those who wish to use the pegging method because it will allow them to recall the mnemonic device in its entirety, without missing any elements.

Chapter 12

Acing Those Exams

> *"Intelligence is the wife, imagination is the mistress, memory is the servant."*
>
> Victor Hugo

This section is dedicated to folks who are having a hard time memorizing details from difficult lessons at school. It doesn't matter what age you are – if you're studying and you need help improving your memory for examinations, this section is definitely for you.

Now, we are going to take a more specific approach to the problem of tough memorizations for school because we're dealing with more material, and the nature of the recall will serve a more complex application.

We are going to make use of earlier strategies and techniques in this section, but we're going lay out the material in such a way that you will be able to go about academic memorization *step-by-step*.

Step 1: Don't just memorize – understand & contextualize

Memorization is often referred to in a negative light because of students who habitually memorize words, phrases and concepts without actually understanding and contextualizing the information.

This is the first challenge to any student who wishes to use memorization as an effective learning tool.

Three parallel processes must run during academic memorization: the rehearsal of information (repetition of chunks of information), *understanding* how the different chunks of information relate to each other and finally, *contextualizing* the information based on the general flow of the subject matter.

If you have been using the 'mechanical' route to memorization, it's time to let go of that method because it rarely helps students pass examinations.

Usually, students who mechanically memorize their notes and books end up being frustrated with exams. They often cannot understand difficult questions because they have not made the proper contextualization and associations between the concepts that they have just memorized.

Ready to do it the right way? Here's how:

1. If you have a slew of notes and diagrams in front of you, *stop*. You need to organize your notes first. Organize your material any way you want, but make sure that the arrangement will provide a logical stream of ideas and concepts.

    If your teacher tends to jump from one topic to another (and this has jumbled your own notes), you can use mini-notes to highlight what topics are contained within specific pages of your notes.

    If you are having a tough time organizing your reading materials, here are some options:

    - Alphabetization

- One group dedicated for "causes" and one group of notes for "effects"

- Several groups of notes based on similarity of topics

- Grouped notes based on importance

- Numbering notes (chronological arrangement)

- One group dedicated to theories & problems and one group of notes for solutions and detailed explanations.

2. After organizing your reading materials in a manner that makes sense to *you*, start reading the various groups of notes. Rephrase and restate the concepts and ideas in your own words.

3. If something confuses you, forget about skipping the topic. The World Wide Web is a 24-hour help area for confused students. Clarify parts of your material through quick research before returning to your initial reading of your review materials. This way, there will be no gaps in your knowledge.

Step 2: Create links and networks of ideas

You can check out the other strategies we have outlined earlier to create memorable associations of ideas. If the pegging method and general mnemonics are inadequate, you can try the *loci* method.

The loci method associates strings of ideas to physical locations.

For example, you can create associations with objects in your room to remember concepts for a particular subject. Once you're done with that subject, you can move on to other physical loci (locations) to memorize facts and concepts from other subjects.

Step 3: The final step

Once you have successfully implemented a mnemonic system for all the materials that you have to study, it's time to *review* all the notes that you have created for yourself. This step will ensure that you will be able to transfer all the knowledge that you have just revisited to your long-term memory.

As we have mentioned earlier, the successful transfer of information from short-term memory to long-term memory requires a minimum of three repetitions, so it would be best if you re-read your notes and revisited your mnemonic images at least three times before calling it a night.

To make your review sessions more effective, here are some tips:

1. If you are an auditory learner, read your notes and mnemonic devices out loud so you can reabsorb the information through hearing. Visual learners, on the other hand, can try scribbling short lists and diagrams to reinforce what you have already read.

2. If you have a portable audio recorder, record your notes and listen to them throughout the day.

3. You can create custom flash cards by simply writing notes on index cards. Buy a large pack of large index cards so you can write down difficult formulas and information easily. Since index cards can easily be reviewed, you will be able to memorize more material more quickly.

Now, reviewing reading materials, notes and mnemonic devices would be much more effective if you reviewed at specific times to achieve specific goals. In the final analysis, the final phase (reviewing) would make up some forty percent of the entire memorization and learning effort.

Time of the Review	Goal
Immediately after the class ends	To fix concepts to your short-term memory
A few hours before sleeping	To help the brain transfer information from the short-term memory center to the long-term memory center
No more than twenty-four hours after the lesson	First reinforcement of material (long-term memory)
Every day after the lesson has been given	Short, continuous reinforcement of material (long-term memory)

30 days after the lesson has been given	Long-term preparation for long examinations

The Truth About Memorization

Memorization and reviewing will only work if you make an effort to consciously build your knowledge on a daily basis.

This applies most especially if the subject at hand involves small bits of information like names, dates and mini- concepts that have to be memorized *within context* to make sense during examinations.

To be on the safe side, it would be best if you dedicate a few minutes every day to scan all your notes and recall information with the use of your mnemonic devices. This is the best way to reinforce what you already know so that recall will be very easy during the actual examination.

Don't forget to *test* all your knowledge before the day of the exam. You can do this in two ways: you can ask questions *or* you can look at specific words/concepts and explain each one using the knowledge you have in store. Try both approaches and see which works for you.

Conclusion

We have covered a lot of territory in this book but hopefully you've gained some understanding about the wonders of memory recall.

Here's a recap of what you've learned:

- The various memory sub-types

- Strategies and exercises to help with memory recall

- Steps to take to beat absentmindedness

- Levels of memory loss

- Tips to help study for exams

Now in order to actually help improve your memory, you'll need to practice some of the techniques you've learned. Make a regular habit of working on memory exercises and you'll be rewarded with sharper recall skills, increased confidence and more satisfaction with your life.

References

Constance, Robin *Your Unlimited Magnificent Memory* (Nebraska: iUniverse) 2005

Culpin, Vicki *Memory Pocketbook* (UK: Management Pocketbooks, Ltd.) 2010

Fotuhi, Majid *The Memory Cure: How to Protect Your Brain Against Memory Loss and Alzheimer's Disease* (New York: McGraw Hill) 20003

Gediman, Corinne *Brainfit: 10 Minutes a Day for a Sharper Mind and Memory* (Tennessee: Routledge Hill Press) 2005

Karges, Craig *Ignite Your Intuition* (Florida: Health Communications, Inc.) 1999

Podder, Tanushree *Smart Memory: Techniques to Improve Memory* (New Delhi: Publishers Pustak Mahal) 2005

Rowan, James *The Missing Memory Link: Programming Verbal Memory* (USA:Lulu Publishing) 2008

Index

A

Absentmindedness 89, 103
Adrenaline 30, 31
Advanced Memory Loss 55, 57, 58
Alphabetization 97
Alzheimer's 25, 40-41, 44, 55, 106
Antioxidants 45
Anxiety 24
Auditory Learner 73, 100

B

B12 Deficiency 44
Bad Cholesterol See LDL
Brain Cells 11
Brain Exercise 69

C

Cholesterol 40, 41, 42, 43
Cholesterol-Memory Connection 40
Cortisol 30, 31

D

Dementia 25
Dietary Fiber 41

E

Early Memory Loss 55-56

F

Folate 47-48

H

Homocysteine 43-44
Human memory 9-12, 15-18, 21-22, 26, 30, 35, 76

L

LDL 40-41
Lipoproteins See Cholesterol,
Loci Method 99
Long-Term Memory 17

M

Memorization 74, 95-96, 102
Memory Cues 92-93
Memory Encoding 17
Mind-Body Connection 39
Mnemonic System 77-78, 80, 99
Mnemonics 75, 76, 81
Mortality Rate 34
Multitasking 24, 35-37, 63, 91

O

Omega-3 42
Organoleptic 66-67
Oxidative Stress 45
Oxygen 11, 30, 31

P

Physical Activity 43, 49, 52

R

Red Wine 43
Repetition 25

S

Sensory 15-17, 49, 67, 74
Sensory Memory 15-17
Short-Term Memory 16
Sleep 31-35, 49
Smoking 42

Statins 41-43
Store Memories 15
Stress 29, 89

T

Tocopherol 48
To Do Lists 19

V

Visual Learners 73
Visualization 27, 92
Vitamins 46-47

Printed in Great Britain
by Amazon